Salt for Horses

Also by Stephanie Krahl

Books

Guiding Principles of Natural Horse Care

Affiliated Websites

www.stephaniekrahl.com
www.soulfulequine.com
www.soulfulcreatures.com
www.soulfulequinebooks.com
www.naturalhorseconcepts.com

Salt for Horses

Tragic Mistakes to Avoid

STEPHANIE KRAHL

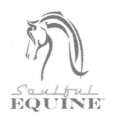

Soulful Creatures™ LLC

ers. All other names are used for identification purposes only and are trademarks or registered trademarks of their respective companies.

This book is dedicated to the real horse lovers who make their choices with intent and promote their horse's health naturally.

Acknowledgments

Martin Krahl
Lynn McKay
G.T. Moore
Mary Tousley
Sharon Tousley

And ...

The Horses of Soulful Equine

CONTENTS

LEGAL INFORMATION

DISCLAIMER

Salt for Horses is for informational and educational purposes only and the contents of this book are protected under freedom of speech and freedom of religion. The information presented and contained within this book is based on the training and experience of the author. Its content is not intended to be used as a substitute for professional medical advice nor is it intended to diagnose, treat, cure, or prevent any disease. **Always** consult a qualified health professional/veterinarian for any medical concerns, questions or advice. The reader assumes all risks from the use, nonuse, or misuse of this information. Neither Stephanie Krahl, Soulful Equine, Soulful Creatures LLC, nor any of their editors, partners, affiliates, or subsidiaries will be held accountable in any way for the use, nonuse, or misuse of the information presented herein or appearing on the Soulful Equine website. While this book is as accurate as the author can make it, there may be unintentional errors, omissions, and inaccuracies.

THE ALL IMPORTANT BOOK MAP

"I don't think much of a man who is not wiser today than he was yesterday."
~ Abraham Lincoln

Did you know that salt plays an important role in your horse's health? Without it, life would not be possible. There are a multitude of misconceptions about feeding salt to horses – many of which I'll cover in this book. Some horse guardians know nothing about this precious subject while others simply select what's on sale at their local feed store. The subject of salt is mentioned in equine circles, and assumptions are made, but for the most part, it's usually glossed over. This is where you're different. Since you care deeply for your horse, I'm confident you won't gloss over the information contained in this book.

The subject of "salt and horses" is an interesting one, and it's necessary for you to understand the role it plays in your equine partner's overall health. Additionally, it's important to know what to avoid when it comes to, what I consider, tragic mistakes when choosing the type of salt to feed your horse.

I'm going to dig deep into the importance of choosing the right kind of salt. Throughout this book I use the terms "refined" and "unrefined" salt.

As you'll learn, although there are many similarities between the two, from a health standpoint they're worlds apart.

To keep it simple, one is highly processed (refined) and the other (unrefined) is closer to what nature intended. As far as these two terms are concerned, I'm going to keep it that simple. There's no need to burden you with more technical details that are not necessary. This is not intended to be a science book. As you proceed you will find that I provide the details for feeding your horse salt, tips and tricks, what to watch out for, the different types of salt you can purchase, and where to purchase your horse's salt products.

Before you begin, find a comfortable place to relax that allows you to absorb the factual data provided. You may be tempted to jump ahead to the sections that give you the details about feeding your horse salt. Do your best to understand the *why* first so you don't feel the need to go with whatever the next horse person you run into recommends.

Knowing the reasons behind why you choose to feed certain foods to your horse is invaluable. In the end, it will help you refrain from prematurely jumping onto the next popular equine product wave simply because you'll be much more informed than the next person.

It is also important to understand that both equine and human nutritionists - in most cases - have a lot of hangups from what they learned in school. Something to think about is this. Have you ever visited someone in the hospital and noticed what they had for lunch or dinner? Rarely have I ever witnessed anything healthy fed to a patient in a hospital. It's usually highly processed, denatured foods that have little or no nutritional value. Some of those foods are known to aggravate and/or cause the actual disease the person is in the hospital for. In other words, dead, processed food is being served to a compromised individual. Those meals are formulated and selected by highly trained nutritionists.

Commercially processed equine feeds, that contain denatured ingredients, are also formulated by highly trained nutritionists – but of the equine variety. So, my point is this, a human or equine nutritionist is usually great at educating about the science of nutrition, but they're usually not capable of promoting health for you or your horse. The reason is that they're closely linked to what is often referred to as "The Sickness Industry." You may have to read between the lines on that insight, but overall I feel you'll easily grasp what I'm sharing with you.

As I mentioned in my book, *Guiding Principles of Natural Horse Care*, one challenge many equine guardians have difficulty overcoming is the "Monkey See, Monkey Do" pattern. Over time you can identify these repetitive patterns in many areas of equine care. When it comes to equine nutrition, a common pattern I've noticed is that an authority figure – usually a popular equine nutritionist - will make a statement about something related to equine nutrition; then somehow it quickly becomes a golden rule. Many times the information provided by these individuals is only partially correct, and sometimes it's completely wrong. Much of this behavior is based on what I call detrimental science versus responsible and ethical scientific progress. A lot of the information taught today by traditionalists does not usually benefit a horse in the long term nor does it benefit your pocket book.

The difficult part of it all is that most people don't know much about promoting their own health let alone what it takes to establish and maintain a naturally healthy horse. Most times their own beliefs and patterns (as it relates to their health and wellness) are reflected directly on to their horse. Usually, those less than ideal patterns are destructive to the horse, and the guardian is often unaware of the consequences. That said, it can be challenging to find valid health information, or even to know where to turn.

My goal is to be your guide, and over time, help you with this challenge. The more you learn, the easier it becomes to weed through the abundance of information we're now exposed to in the Internet age. I'll share with you key principles that will save you a significant amount of time doing your research. Eventually you'll become a lot like a coffee filter – only allowing the good stuff to get through.

My personal belief is that the better you under-stand what it takes for you to stay healthy and prevent disease, the easier it is to filter through the information that's not in your horse's best interest. What I'll share with you about salt also relates to your own health, so I'd recommend you pursue further education regarding this subject using the resources I provide at the end of this book.

HISTORY, FACTS AND LEGENDS

"If you don't know history, then you don't know anything. You are a leaf that doesn't know it is part of a tree."
~ Michael Crichton

Salt has a remarkable history within many cultures including the ancient Hebrews, Greeks, Romans and Chinese. Having salt readily available - as we do today - is a luxury. European kings and Egyptian pharaohs would have been amazed at this availability. Now we can access high quality salts from all over the world easily through the Internet. We are living in the best time ever where we have such access to *any* high quality food we choose to investigate and try.

Salt: A World History by Mark Kurlansky contains amazing stories about our most precious commodity, salt. The earliest writing about salt dates back to around 800 B.C. in China. For centuries, Chinese governments saw salt as a source of state revenue. In China, writings were discovered that mentioned a salt tax had existed in the twentieth century B.C. Since salt is a necessary substance for survival and good health, it made an excellent tax generator because everyone had to have it. Salt was also used to pay the Roman army. It was as good as gold!

A factoid: Salt is the origin of the word "salary," derived from the fact that the Roman soldiers were paid in salt. Eventually, this came to signify a stipend paid in any form, usually money. Today if you're working hard and earning your salary you are said to be "worth your salt."

Some of the earliest Egyptian burial sites date from around 3000 B.C. Ancient Egyptians used salt to embalm bodies. Without salt, there would have been no mummies. An interesting bit of history: the Egyptians would place preserved foods in a tomb of the the deceased. They believed that the person who passed needed to be well-equipped for their journey to the afterlife. Not only were bodies well-preserved, but tombs contained preserved food offerings. Most offerings included jars of salt, vegetables, fruits, fish, and meat.

Traveling to the afterlife was believed to be a long journey, therefore the deceased's body and the food offerings needed to be preserved in order to withstand the trip. The Egyptians understood salt's essential value because it was believed to make the death passage possible. It is thought that the Egyptians were the first to cure meat and fish with salt. They certainly were the first civilization to preserve foods with salt on a large scale. Salt keeps food from going bad by drawing out moisture which can cause bacteria to grow. It can also help to kill bacteria. This discovery was another reason salt was considered an invaluable substance since in those times, there was no refrigeration.

The healing powers of salt were recognized by Hippocrates - an ancient Greek physician (born in 460 B.C.). He recommended many salt remedies for healing various health issues such as infections and clearing congestion, to name but two. Although Hippocrates is credited and known for many accomplishments as it relates to medicine, most people will recall two things – the coining of the Hippocratic Oath and a notable quote especially popular in health and wellness fields:

"Let food be thy medicine and medicine be thy food" ~ Hippocrates

The meaning and power of this quote is often forgotten in our modern times *especially* by westerners.

As you can see, salt's rich history has shaped us as human beings. However, salt's recent history leaves a lot to be desired. It's thought of by most to be an enemy rather than a mineral that nourishes and heals the body. Salt has developed into something much different than what nature intended. Now it's mass produced and refined. This mass production has resulted in the use of toxic chemicals and other unnatural agents that are harmful to you and your equine partner.

Processed (refined) table salt is a harmful additive

that when consumed in excess and over time has been shown to have an adverse effect on health. Refinement of salt completely erases any healthful benefits and consuming it leaves you or your equine partner susceptible to a variety of health problems. Processed table salt is in most everything – pet food, baby food, potato chips, canned goods, etc. It's in most anything processed.

SALT AND HOW IT RELATES TO HEALTH

"It's bizarre that the produce manager is more important to my children's health than the pediatrician." ~ Meryl Streep

ALL ANIMALS AND HUMANS REQUIRE SALT

Salt is just as important as needing air to breathe and it's necessary for sustaining life on this planet. All mammals - including humans – must eat sodium chloride (a scientific name for salt) in order to live.

If you recall any of the medical drama shows or reality shows you've watched on TV, you'll remember that one of the first things they often do when someone is in an emergency situation is place them on an I.V. of saline solution. That's because saline is the safest fluid to give quickly in large volumes. The adult human body is made up of approximately 70%

water and roughly 250 grams of salt and the two are necessary for the optimal functioning of the hormonal, nervous, digestive and immune systems as well as for metabolism, detoxification and the transportation of nutrients.[1] Blood is about 0.9% salt, 77% of it is sodium chloride, with smaller amounts of potassium, calcium, and bicarbonate.[2] This isn't just true for humans but is true for all vertebrate animals. The body is like the ocean because its fluids closely resemble sea water. The similarities between our bodies and the ocean are fascinating. One of the most important things needed for the body is a high quality living salt that contains vital minerals the body needs – this holds true for you and your horse.

Those in agriculture know how important salt is and often provide it in the form of salt blocks or "licks." What many people don't know is how critical it is that their salt is in an unrefined form versus refined for both humans and animals. Some people believe that salt is toxic and isn't good for the body, but most all creatures require living salt and it is essential for health.

High quality unrefined salts are alkaline forming, because all the minerals are still intact. These unrefined salts are between 80 and 90% sodium chloride with additional trace minerals, but table salt is close to 99% sodium chloride and it has been refined to the point where the minerals have been striped out. The remaining percentage no longer consists of trace minerals. Instead, it consists of chemical additives. Without the naturally occurring minerals intact, salt is highly *acid forming*. No one wants that for their horse. We already have enough problems with the common occurrence of ulcers in horses. As you'll soon learn in the pages before you, the downsides to you consuming refined salt or feeding it to your horse, are many.

THE QUALITY OF YOUR SALT MATTERS

Technically, all salt comes from the sea, whether it's from oceans millions of years ago that are now trapped under the earth or from today's oceans. What matters from a health standpoint is how that salt is harvested, where it comes from, and how it's processed. Most people don't give the quality of the salt they're consuming or the salt they feed their horse a second thought. This state of mind, and the manner in which you act on that information, can cause serious health consequences later down the road for you and your horse.

In *The All Important Book Map* section, I briefly defined the two terms you need to be aware of as they relate to salt – refined and unrefined. One additional term to understand is "living salt." To keep it simple, you ideally want to consume and feed your horse what's called a living salt (more on that to come). Living salt is also unrefined, and in the form nature intended. Refined salt is less than ideal and I consider it a toxic substance. This is usually what you see sitting on the table at your local restaurant. You probably have it in your cupboard. It's also what is used as a preservative in a large portion of processed foods in America today.

From a quality standpoint, the first step is to understand there *is* a difference when it comes to choosing salt. Quality matters! If it's a refined, toxic table salt, this is a poor quality choice. If it's an unrefined, whole food salt, this is the best choice.

SALT IS SALT, IS SALT ... OF COURSE IT'S NOT

TYPICAL INDUSTRIAL STYLE TABLE SALT

Most people are only familiar with refined salt (white table salt) that comes out of the typical salt shaker, and some people feed that same salt to their horse. However, there's an abundance of different types of natural, healthy salts. Just like any other product you purchase, salt quality varies and so do your options. The purpose of this section is to focus on the differences between two essential terms – refined and unrefined salt.

When salt is in its natural form it's called unrefined salt. Unrefined salt is not manipulated or reshaped by man. It's as close as possible to the form Mother Nature intended. When it's not chemically processed and altered, salt contains many elements and minerals needed by the body. These minerals also act as a buffer so salt will have an alkalizing effect on the body versus an acidifying effect. Acidity promotes disease rather than health. When key natural minerals are removed - as it is when salt is refined - salt becomes acidic. Refined salt lacks the buffering effect of the other minerals which is why it's acidifying to the body. Cancer and chronic illness are two consequences of an acidic pH. To drive this point home, pure water is said to have a neutral pH (close to 7.0). Celtic Sea Salt® (which is one unrefined salt option) has been shown to increase the pH of water, thereby making it less acidic while refined salt has been shown to decrease the pH, making it more acidic.[3] Therefore, the best salt to choose for optimal health is unrefined.

Mother Nature knew what she was doing when she created natural salts for us. It's wise not to mess that up. However, man often comes along and thinks he can improve on Mother Nature. This is why over time the fear has been programmed into society that salt is bad. This fear is the result of the toxic chemical industry. That fear is warranted if you consume or feed your horse refined salt. What's bad is that refined salt contains toxic substances the body attempts to manage and flush out of the system. In the meantime, this refined salt causes health problems.

As I stated in the section *History, Facts, and Legends*, processed table salt is in most everything – pet food, baby food, potato chips, canned goods, you name it. Now that it's hidden in most everything, the result has been a dramatic increase in salt related health issues and disease.

Since the 1920s there's been a dramatic increase in the manufacturing and use of toxic chemicals. Those chemicals, along with more cost effective methods of harvesting, are used when refining salt. Prior to the 1920s, most of the salt harvested was natural salt which contained essential minerals including the trace mineral iodine.[4] Throughout history, salt making was considered an art. In current times it has been degraded to a business solely based on profit, not on promoting the health of our civilization.

Refined table salts are collected from sea water (often from not-so-pristine locales such as the South San Francisco Bay) or harvested from underground salt mines. After water-flushing, table salt manufacturers will typically treat and remove unwanted elements (translated mostly to mean "needed minerals") using chemical agents such as barium, sulfuric acid and chlorine (yes, chlorine is bad for you). The resulting product is dried at more than 1,200 degrees Fahrenheit, and tainted with toxic chemicals. Since all the moisture is taken out of salt when it's refined, it has the tendency to clump. To keep this from happening, anti-caking agents are added. They prevent salt from mixing with water and also prevent salt from doing one of its most important functions in the body, which is regulating hydration.[5]

These chemical agents are often aluminum based. What's used is either sodium aluminosilicate or sodium ferrocyanide in quantities as high as 13 parts per million.[6] It's common knowledge that aluminum has been found to cause health issues in humans. For example, aluminum has been linked to Alzheimer's. These anti-caking substances make it difficult for the body to properly utilize and absorb the salt.

In the United States, corn syrup (see the resources section for additional information) is usually added as a binder for iodine and to possibly help cover-up the bitterness of refined salt.[7] If you haven't read my article, *Are You Feeding Your Horse These 4 'Healthy' – Yet Dangerous – Foods?* (see the resources section), you may want to. I go into great detail on the dangers of feeding corn products to horses. It doesn't matter what form of corn you feed, corn oil, corn syrup, whole corn, processed corn, etc.

Other additives to industrial refined iodized table salt are substances such as calcium oxide and calcium carbonate to increase salt's whiteness. Synthetic forms of calcium are considered "bad calcium" sources, because they've been linked to calcification of the body that is the result of excess calcium buildup. Most all calcium on the market today that's contained in supplements (and that's added to refined and processed products) is made from chalk – this is not a good source of calcium. What you want to consume and to feed your horse is calcium that's digestible and that naturally occurs in whole foods.

Many refined salt manufacturers add iodine. If you're worried about your horse getting adequate amounts of iodine, the amount added to refined salt is inadequate for the body's needs. In humid conditions,

most of the iodine evaporates anyway the longer iodized refined salt sits on the shelf. Therefore, with time,
iodine levels will decrease in these refined, iodized
table salt products. Iodine from natural unrefined salt
is utilized and tolerated better by the body. A quality
unrefined sea salt, such as Celtic Sea Salt, contains
more natural iodine per gram (approximately 150 mcg)
than your typical iodized table salt (approximately 50-
80 mcg).[8] It is important to ensure your horse is getting adequate amounts of iodine, however, there are
much better alternatives than feeding iodized table
salt.

Table salt is a highly processed form of sodium
chloride sometimes with added iodine. There's nothing
natural about it and it's loaded with toxic chemicals.
Something to consider about refined salt is that all
the important minerals that nature intended for us to
consume have been extracted by the refined salt
industry to be used in the chemical industry. As an
example, magnesium is removed prior to selling the
refined salt to you for consumption. The reason?
There are many, but the main one is that the selling of
these "extracted" minerals is much more profitable to
the refined salt industry than selling whole food form
salt to you.

Refined salt can cause abnormal function throughout your horse's body and disrupt balance. For example,
if you feed standard table salt to your horse, you're
causing an imbalance in your horse's system between
the different types of electrolytes (sodium, potassium,
magnesium, and chloride). Electrolytes are important

for circulation, muscle contraction, and nerve function.

I know that many equine experts recommend feeding loose iodized table salt to your horse. Based on my research and experience, feeding your horse refined table salt is not the best choice and is a tragic mistake in my book. This is one way horse guardians are unintentionally introducing additional toxins into their horse's body. This is one toxic substance you have control over, so it's best to choose a better option than refined table salt.

COMMON TABLE SALT PLOYS

Some experts state that salt is a chemical - so why should you be concerned about the "other chemicals" used to refine salt? What's important is to distinguish the difference between a safe chemical substance and one that is a hazardous substance.

To say the chemicals used in refined salt processing are the same as those naturally occurring chemical compounds in unrefined salt is inappropriate and inaccurate. Comparing all chemicals and saying they're the same is not rational. This is one way people justify their stance and try to convince you that it's okay that toxic substances are added to and used in the salt refining process.

Have you ever seen the movie *Erin Brockovich* starring Julia Roberts? If you haven't, now is a good time to watch it so my point will become more clear. This film is a true story of Erin Brockovich who fought against an energy corporation called Pacific Gas and Electric Company (PG&E). In short, PG&E was poisoning the water supply of a small town in Hinkley, California. Remember, this is a true story! Over time, many people in that town developed various forms of terminal cancer. The medical doctors hired by PG&E convinced an entire town that the PG&E by-product that was contaminating their water supply was "good for them." What PG&E intentionally claimed was good for the town's people was instead a highly hazardous, carcinogenic substance called hexavalent chromium.[9]

Straight up chromium is a mineral we're all familiar with and we know it's good for us in the appropriate form and amount. However, hexavalent chromium is produced in industrial processes and is known to cause cancer. The safest form of chromium to consume is in whole foods. For example, cinnamon is a good source of chromium. Who doesn't love cinnamon? Plus, it's good for you because your body uses chromium in small amounts for normal function. It's known to help move blood sugar (glucose) from the bloodstream into the cells and to turn fats, carbohydrates, and proteins into energy.[10]

So yes, in chemistry, technically both forms of chromium described above can be called "chemicals," but as you can clearly see, one is safe and the other is quite hazardous. PG&E was telling the town they were using a safe form of chromium, when instead they were using a toxic form. This is an excellent example of where innocent people blindly believed a medical doctor who told them the hexavalent chromium was *not* causing the outbreak of cancer in their town. The same is true with table salt – sodium chloride is the major chemical compound present (generally safe), but other chemicals like barium, sulfuric acid, and chlorine (generally considered toxic) are used in processing table salt.

This type of stuff goes on frequently. What I described to you is a common pattern when it comes to industrialization and unethical companies who don't care about you or the health of your horse. It's not always wise to listen to someone just because they have a lot of letters after their name. And money isn't *always* the motivator of someone making such statements that cause harm. Ignorance or reluctance to think on their own is often to blame and the harm they create is usually unintentional. However, keep this in mind, much of Western medicine would be more appropriately called the "sickness industry" instead of the "health industry." Individuals who enter those "health industry" professions with the best of intentions are usually educated by the very people who have a lot to gain by keeping you or your horse sick.

MOTHER NATURE'S SALT

Unrefined salt, which I like to call "Mother Nature's Salt," is a safe and natural holistic remedy. Pure (in this context, the word "pure" implies a food whose essence has not been changed by processing or additives) unrefined natural sea salt is rich in minerals and natural electrolytes which are necessary for optimal health. Other than sodium and chloride, unrefined salt contains over 80 essential minerals, where as refined salt contains none. Unrefined salt contains all the minerals it originally possessed such as magnesium and potassium which are essential for a healthy immune system. There are no toxic additives. It's a whole food product that's easily utilized by the body.

An unrefined salt such as Celtic Sea Salt is considered a "living salt" and it's more living than rock salt (Himalayan pink salt which is unrefined). Living salts are also more bio-available to the body and they contain high concentrations of Ormus minerals, which are more important to life in general than "trace minerals." Ormus minerals are atoms that do not fit into the Mendeleev's Periodic Table of Elements or Walter Russell's Periodic Chart.[11]

"Dead salt" and "living salt" is an important idea. Salt lives! It has a life force. The concept is much like living food and dead food. You want to consume and feed a living salt because it is the best choice for your horse's health and for your health.

Something to consider, Himalayan salt (and other unrefined rock salts) has been under the earth for a long time. It's much further away from the life force – the ocean. Where as unrefined sea salts are closer to the life force. Therefore, when you put them in water, they're much more bio-available. What you'll want to do is experiment with different salts and see what's best for your horse and for you. The most important principle to take away is to avoid refined salt and be careful when it comes to clever marketing or anyone who recommends that you feed your horse refined table salt.

REASONS WHY SALT IS PROCESSED

So why would manufacturers go to the trouble to refine salt?

According to Dr. Brownstein in his book *Salt Your Way to Health*, there are four reasons:

➢ To help assure a long shelf life
➢ To ensure the resulting product is all white - manufacturers believe it looks cleaner
➢ To remove the toxins, if it was taken from a polluted area
➢ To add iodine to prevent goiter (read Dr Brownstein's book *Iodine, Why You Need It, Why You Can't Live Without It*)

So not only have so many of the natural, whole food form minerals our bodies crave been removed, but other toxic chemicals have been added. Additionally, dextrose (sugar) has been added to cover up the bad tastes left behind by these chemicals - something many diabetics are not aware of.

You can taste the difference between unrefined salt and table salt. It *is* obvious. A fun exercise you may want to try – ask some of the best chefs what kind of salt they use for cooking their wonderful creations. I feel confident the answer you won't hear is "table salt." Chefs take great pride in their food creations and usually seek out the best natural salts to season with. Try switching to unrefined salt yourself and taste the difference. Your body knows best.

> *"Common, refined table salt is bitter, metallic, and overly-salty - not at all the kind of palatal experience natural salt provides. Refined salt also has pushed the whole of salt to villain status in our modern times. Unhealthy, unnecessary, and unwholesome - we have grown to fear salt."* [12]

NATURAL ENVIRONMENTAL EFFECTS ON SALT

Any salt that is made by the evaporation of sun and wind is subject to the effects of the environment. These effects can include such things as birds, algae, pollens, etc. One concern some people express is for the pollution that exists in the sea. No oceans in today's world are unaffected by pollution. Should this be a concern? Yes and no. It's all relative.

To put things in perspective, let me remind you how refined salt is made. It's made with chemical agents such as barium, sulfuric acid, chlorine, anti-caking chemicals, dextrose, and sometimes even fluoride. Additionally, it strips away all the beneficial minerals the body so desperately needs which also causes acidifying effects. Without the minerals there's no buffer to prevent acidity.

So no, comparatively, it's not a concern. Additionally, everything is polluted – you can't get away from it. What you can do is choose the cleanest sources you have access to and choose whole food substances, such as unrefined salt. In this day and age, we have abundance at our fingertips, literally. In the age of the Internet, you can easily gain access to high quality food sources for your equine partner, yourself and for the rest of your family. You can also seek out the cleanest sources available rather than resorting to supporting the chemical and sickness industries because it's convenient. One caveat I'd like to add: I believe that when you support such industries or individuals who promote those industries, there is a karmic effect. It effects *your* karma. If you believe in karma, as I do, then it's something to consider. If you don't believe in karma, it still matters because the actions you take today come back around to effect you one way or another in the future – good or bad.

KEY POINTS ABOUT SALT DIFFERENCES AND HEALTH

By now, you have fully grasped the importance of choosing the right kind of salt so you can promote your horse's health and yours. Below are some bullet points for easy reference on the differences between refined (bad and unhealthy) and unrefined (Mother Nature's creation full of health promoting goodness) salt.

Refined Salt:

Based on the information I provided previously in this book, below are a few key points to fully grasp regarding the issues with refined salt:

- ➢ Many of the minerals our bodies require and crave have been removed.
- ➢ Toxic chemicals have been added.
- ➢ Dextrose (sugar) and/or corn syrup have been added to cover up the bad tastes left behind by the chemicals used to process salt. Something many diabetics are not aware of (what about insulin resistant horses?)
- ➢ It's lacking the buffering effect of the minerals and is acidifying to the body, which can cause chronic disease as well as inflammation. Think about horses who have issues with ulcers – this is a common concern.
- ➢ It is not a whole food product and, therefore, cannot be easily utilized by the body.
- ➢ It has a bitter, metallic, and overly salty taste.

Unrefined Salt:

Now, let's have a look at some key points about unrefined salt.

- ➢ It contains all the minerals it originally possessed such as magnesium and potassium which are essential for a healthy immune system.
- ➢ There are no toxic additives.
- ➢ No sugar is added.
- ➢ The naturally occurring minerals are not chemically removed and they provide a buffering effect,

so acidity is not an issue.

➢ It's a whole food product that's easily utilized by the body where the naturally occurring minerals are in proper balance, including needed trace and Ormus minerals.

➢ Iodine from unrefined salt is utilized and tolerated better by the body.

➢ A high quality unrefined sea salt, such as Celtic Sea Salt, contains more natural iodine per gram (approximately 150 mcg) than your typical iodized table salt (approximately 50-80 mcg).

➢ Natural, unrefined salt tastes wonderful – it is nothing like refined table salt.

VETERINARIAN OR DOCTOR RECOMMENDED

The doctor of the future will give no medication, but will interest his patients in the care of the human frame, diet and in the cause and prevention of disease.
~ Thomas A. Edison

With every so called fact there will be an opposing view. At that point, you have to use your best judgment, common sense, and intuition. One of my favorite quotes is by Dr. Joesph Mercola:

"Sometimes common sense trumps empirical evidence."

As with many subjects in the nutrition and medical industries, when it comes to using or not using a refined salt, this is an excellent statement. The problem with that statement is that if common sense was so common more people would have it. I feel the biggest problem with the decisions we make when it comes to our health or the health of our horses, is that we have to get out of our head, into our heart, and make way for our intuition.

I usually don't condone the phrase "doctor recommended" or "veterinarian recommended" unless it comes from more conscious individuals who are not trapped by conventional thinking. You can easily identify these people.

Below are a few examples of what *unconventional* doctors are saying about using unrefined salts such as Celtic Sea Salt®, Redmond Real Salt®, or Himilayan Sea Salt:

> "Many illnesses are caused or exacerbated by trace-mineral deficiencies. These can be avoided by the liberal use of Celtic Sea Salt® in your cooking and the complete avoidance of all other salts, all of which contain only pure sodium chloride." ~ Dr. Thomas S. Cowan, M.D.[13]

> "Standard table salt upsets the balance and causes abnormal function throughout your body." ~ Mark Force, DC[14]

> "Refined salt lacks minerals and causes acidosis (i.e., a lowered pH). Our bodies were meant to function optimally with adequate mineral levels and adequate salt intake. Only the use of unrefined salt can provide both of these factors." ~ Dr. David Brownstein, M.D.[15]

If you've noticed throughout this book, I refer often to Dr. David Brownstein, M.D. on the subject of salt. He's considered one of the pioneers in this area of health and wellness.

I could include in this book opposing statements by some popular equine nutritionists who consistently recommend feeding refined, iodized table salt to your horse. However, it's not worth my time or your time. What I will state is this: I liken the recommendation of feeding refined salt to your horse to a medical doctor telling a patient not to take vitamin D3 or that it's not an important nutrient. This happens, believe it or not. In my eyes, that recommendation should be considered malpractice because vitamin D3 is the most powerful molecule found. Vitamin D3 turns on more genes that express healing and health than any other single substance that we currently know of.[16] The important take-away is to identify those individuals who recommend feeding refined table salt to your horse and make it a point to not take that advice.

A common occurrence is that some things may sound ridiculous at first, but in the end, proven to be correct. My simple rule of thumb is to not take something at face value, especially when it's coming from a conventional establishment. Most theories are just that, theories, and don't work in the real world or are tainted by unethical companies who couldn't care less about your or your horse's health.

A good principle to consider is to explore the opposite of what everyone else does, thinks, or believes (which usually stems from conventional wisdom or so-called experts). From personal experiences in both my own health journey and with that of my horses, I often find that it is in questioning conventional wisdom that I discover valid answers and approaches that achieve positive results. This principle has proven to me, over and over, to be consistently correct.

WHAT THE EQUINE EXPERTS DON'T TELL YOU

"Any intelligent fool can make things bigger, more complex, and more violent. It takes a touch of genius – and a lot of courage – to move in the opposite direction."
~ Albert Einstein

One of the first things you probably learned about horses is that you need to make sure you provide them a salt lick or loose table salt. Free choice is ideal. You may have even been told to avoid whole food forms of salt which contain naturally occurring minerals. Some experts believe that these whole food forms of salt may contain too much of a particular mineral or will cause you issues "balancing" your horse's diet. There are many misconceptions about feeding salt to horses.

It's common for someone to drive down to their local feed store and purchase a chemically processed, large, white, hardened salt block for their livestock. It's also common for some experts to recommend that you feed your horse the refined loose iodized table salt that you may have sitting on your kitchen table right now. Neither of these solutions is ideal for your horse. Not only are they less than ideal, but over time they may cause health issues as discussed previously.

Many may argue that refined iodized table salt will not cause problems for horses as it does people. First off, I believe this is an incorrect statement. I've heard the argument on multiple occasions that horses are not like people. I agree with that to a point. However, when we start seeing changes in our environment, or when disease starts to crop up more and more, where do we often see it first? We'll see subtle signs in our animal population. Some signs may not be so subtle, and some animals often mirror what's going on in our human population. An example is the epidemic of human diabetes and obesity which is similar to insulin resistance in horses, frequently leading to laminitis.

The point is, if we can control the amount of toxins and inappropriate and unnatural substances that go into our horses, then why not do it? Salt is only one of many of these substances we can control. I've often heard this statement from government agencies, and also from people who regularly work with toxic chemicals:

"The amount of the toxic chemical in the product is not enough to cause harm to you or your animals."

If this were the case, then it's less likely we'd have

the epidemic of health problems and disease we have today. Large umbrella terms are often used to summarize the results of negative external effects on the body. You don't usually hear the nightly news reporting on the direct effects of aluminum poisoning, mercury poisoning, air pollution, etc. Instead you hear them talk about Alzheimer's, autism, lung cancer, and so on. This is brilliant manipulation.

Brainwashing and greed usually win unless you learn to choose wisely and *un-learn* a lot of what you've been taught. What's not understood is that it's not just a single occurrence you should be concerned about, but rather the cumulative effect of every encounter with "small" toxic substances which you and your horse come in contact with daily. Your everyday choices matter to your health, your family's health, your horse's health, to the environment, and to our future on this planet.

You may think, "Why should I be concerned about feeding my horse a little refined table salt?" A little table salt won't be the only thing that will cause harm to your horse, but it's part of a cumulative effect of everything else your horse is exposed to. The more you can decrease exposure to negative environmental influences, the more you can stack the odds in your horse's favor.

Any time you can minimize toxins and inappropriate and unnatural substances in your horse's diet and environment, then do it. This is especially important if you have a compromised horse, such as one with Cushing's disease, insulin resistance (IR) or equine protozoal myeloencephalitis (EPM), allergies, ulcers, just to name a few.

FINAL THOUGHTS AND OBSERVATIONS

CHOOSE SALT PRODUCTS WISELY

It is well documented that refined salt is not the best choice for optimal health. Refined salt is a chemical experiment, which is not what the body needs or wants. However, unrefined salt has proven to be effective in maintaining optimal health, and it contains every mineral the body needs. It's the best mineral supplement there is and it always has been. We tend to forget that important piece of information. In Dr. David Brownstein's book *Salt Your Way to Health*, he states:

> *"Unrefined salt, containing over 80 minerals, is the perfect source of salt for the body. It provides a proper balance of nutrients that the body can use. My clinical experience has clearly shown that refined salt is not a healthful substance for the body*

and its continued use will lead to the onset of chronic illness." [17]

It's evident that feeding your horse refined salt can lead to health problems in the long-run. Over time, the use of refined foods - such as refined salts - can deplete minerals the body needs to function optimally not to mention the additional toxins consumed. If your horse consistently ingests refined salt, it can lead to thyroid dysfunction, poorly functioning adrenal glands, hormonal problems, and mineral deficiencies. These types of imbalances happen over a period of time; therefore it's easy for most horse guardians to give little thought to the act of feeding refined salt to their horse. On the other side of the coin, unrefined sea salt provides the necessary minerals needed to nourish your horse's body. The well-balanced array of minerals contained in unrefined salt is what's needed for thyroid and other endocrine glands to function in an optimal manner. Unrefined salt should be the salt of choice for a properly functioning equine endocrine system and for overall health.

It's important to get the right kind of salt in your horse's body. Most horse guardians will have to do the "salt switch" and upgrade from feeding a toxic salt (such as loose iodized table or chemical block salts) to a living unrefined sea salt. Although rock salts like Himalayan salt have a multitude of health benefits, I'm a big fan of "living" sea salt. Some think that Himalayan salt is sea salt. It's not. It is rock salt but it is unrefined, which is good. Himalayan salt is rich in minerals. Sea salt is, too, but it has four times more of those minerals. One example of a "living" sea salt is Celtic Sea Salt.

When you start to consume unrefined sea salt yourself, you'll find it's strong in flavor, therefore, you may not need to use as much as refined table salt. Unrefined salt is also nutrient rich and, as with horses, some people find they heavily crave it once they start consuming it and, after a while, they tapper down their consumption. This is usually an indication that the body needs the minerals provided by unrefined salt and that an imbalance exists. Unrefined salt will replenish the body's mineral balance. This is great information you can apply to your equine partner's diet. You can also try it for yourself. In-fact, I'd like to encourage you to do the "salt switch" and gradually detox your body of the toxic salt you may already be consuming.

The most important take away from this information is that the *right kind of salt* is required for health. Unrefined sea salt is the best choice when feeding salt to your equine partner or to your family. Read on for more information about some of the different types of unrefined salt and how it relates to your equine partner.

WHAT DOES ALL THIS MEAN TO YOU AND YOUR ANIMALS?

Use *unrefined* salt, only. Refined/table salt is an inferior choice and you sure don't want to feed it to your horse. Keep in mind that, as of today, it is unlikely you'll hear about feeding unrefined salt from a traditional equine nutritionist, veterinarian, or your doctor. In the equine world, they discuss the benefits of salt but still recommend toxic refined table salt. Doctors tell you to decrease salt intake, which is true if everything you're eating is processed and you still buy table salt. Otherwise, unrefined salt is considered therapeutic. Holistic practitioners have recognized salt as a simple, safe, and effective approach to health for quite some time. It is still not recognized in traditional equine circles of health care. Take recommendations from such sources with a grain of salt (pun intended).

Listed below are the most popular types of unrefined salt fed to horses and used by health-conscious people. There are countless unrefined salts available other than the ones I've listed below, so I'd like to encourage you to study and try others. One salt I listed in this section - Icelandic Flake Salt - may be a little pricy to feed to your horse, but you may want to consider trying it yourself.

Celtic Sea Salt® brand is an authentic, unprocessed whole therapeutic salt that comes from the coastline of Brittany France. Since 1976 Celtic Sea Salt has been harvested using a method that preserves the purity and balance of ocean minerals. The Light Grey Celtic® is totally unprocessed and hand harvested. It's dried by the sun and the wind, retaining the ocean's moisture and locking in a vast array of vital trace elements. It's a coarse, moist salt that gets a light grey hue from the pure clay sole it's harvested from. The fact that it retains a natural balance of essential minerals (shown by analysis to be 80+) and contains no additives are obvious benefits. Although there are many other wonderful unrefined salts, Celtic is unmatched in flavor. I personally add it to water first thing in the morning or to one of my elixir drinks. It's no surprise that Celtic Sea Salt is highly recommended by many health care practitioners. This is also my salt of choice that I feed daily to my horses.

Redmond Real Salt® comes from the small town of Redmond, in central Utah, approximately 200 miles south of Salt Lake City. The salt is extracted from deep within the earth where it was formed millions of years ago when that part of North America was covered by oceans. Over millions of years the sea water evaporated and at some point during the Jurassic era, a range of volcanoes erupted around the ancient sea bed, sealing the salt with thick volcanic ash, protecting it against the pollution man would eventually introduce into the environment. This salt is produced without additives, chemicals or heat processing. It still includes all the minerals it originally possessed, shown by analysis to be more than 60 natural trace minerals, including iodine.

Himalayan Crystal Salt™ comes from a mine in the Karakorum Range of the Himalayan Mountains in Pakistan. This mine is said to be 200-250 million years old and the salt is still harvested by hand by local traditional miners. It is then hand-selected, hand-crushed, hand-washed and sun-dried. Since this salt is crystalline in nature, it is said to manifest a superior structure and, as such, its elements are supposedly more biochemically available to the cells of animals. Since it comes from deep within the ground, pollution is not a concern.

Icelandic Flake Salt is an artisan salt that's produced with 100% geothermal energy. This is an excellent salt made in an environmentally sustainable manner. It's produced using only energy from geothermal hot springs in the northwest of Iceland. This salt contains 3 times more magnesium and 2 times more potassium than Celtic Sea Salt.

TIPS FOR FEEDING SALT TO YOUR HORSE

I personally like all the salts I've listed in the previous section and consistently feed at least one of them to my horses. For many years I've used Celtic, Redmond's, and Himalayan salt in my own kitchen and still do. My two favorites for horses are Redmond's and Celtic. I like Himalayan salt as well, but I found that the licks didn't hold up well in the humid Texas weather. Usually the smallest amount of rain or humidity would cause them to melt. I think the biggest challenge is the humidity here in Texas. Of course you may find a way around that by feeding Himalayan salt in granular/loose form.

The way I feed salt to my horses is both free choice and with their ration. I feed one heaping tablespoon of Celtic Sea Salt twice per day. This is a good maintenance dose for a 1000 pound horse. During our hot days of summer in Texas I may increase it just a little because horses often need more nutrients in severe heat and the unrefined sea salt also provides additional electrolytes. However, I usually don't increase it much over one tablespoon twice per day. I also provide a free choice Redmond's salt lick in their paddock. The Redmond's licks tend to hold up in the elements. I make sure I put it in a container at ground level that also has drainage holes in the bottom. You can usually find one of these containers at your local feed store. The one I have is often used for the large, square mineral blocks that are purchased for cattle. It works well for my Redmond's Rock.

The reason I don't leave the Celtic Sea Salt out for free choice is because it also doesn't hold up to the Texas elements well. Additionally, I have one horse who loves to play with most everything and tends to dump over any bucket he can find, including water troughs if they get too low. I could find a way around that by bolting a trough down, but because he's so willful, he finds a way to play with most anything. Your situation may be different. If you can, I would recommend leaving out loose salt and the rock lick but also add loose salt to their daily ration. I'm a big believer in providing your horse a lot of variety, so using more than one of the salts I mentioned is a good strategy.

Most people will argue that a horse can't get enough salt from a lick, and that may be true to a point (another half truth). If your horse is extremely deficient in minerals, you shouldn't be attempting to "fix" those severe imbalances with a single salt lick in the first place. Instead, it should be a component of a well rounded natural horse care program.

Something to consider, if a horse is so deficient in minerals and salt, an advantage of a salt lick is that it will slow down their consumption. Otherwise, by providing a severely deficient horse free choice loose salt they may over consume it. Almost anything in excess is not good. Many horses will lick on salt rocks when they need it. Mine don't lick on them often because their diet is rich in whole food nutrients and they get a consistent ration of unrefined sea salt. However, I've had natural hoof care client's horses almost devour Himalayan salt licks as soon as one is put in their pen, which means they were very deficient in minerals - not a good thing.

Here is something to think about - animals in the wild, including horses, are known for seeking out minerals from rock sources. They paw at these sources with their hooves which is another way nature helps shape the hoof. Not only do these rocks provide vital nutrition, but a horse will grind those rocks with their teeth. This is one way nature assists the horse with her dental work by getting rid of the annoying sharp edges.[18] I've never heard of an equine dentist servicing horses in wild horse country, have you? For the domesticated horse, this natural behavior is interpreted by most equine experts as a horse not being able to get enough salt or minerals because the block is chewed on. This type of behavior more than likely has been going on since before equines were domesticated.

Another note on rock salt. The unrefined salt I'm recommending to you is not the same as what you would typically buy at your local feed store that comes in a block form. I grew up on a cattle farm and we used those same types of blocks all the time. Their intended use has always been for cattle and then people started using them for horses. However, horses have a different tongue than cattle – it's much softer versus rough like a cows. A concern is usually raised that these blocks are not made for horses and are not the optimal choice. I agree with that statement, however, I still choose to provide a free-choice Redmond's Rock or Himalayan rock salt. These two rock forms are not in the same league as your typical processed, toxic salt block. There's no comparison. Additionally, both rock salts are generally considered smoother than a traditional salt or mineral block made for cattle.

I also know that Redmond's Rock is used extensively for deer. I would imagine that deer probably have even softer tongues than horses. From my observations and research, deer love Redmond's Rock. If you think logically about this, since the beginning of time animals usually had to get their salt from some rock form. So my point is that all this concern and talk about using a block versus not using one is valid – but it's only valid in a traditional salt "block" sense. Use your best judgment as far as using a free choice unrefined salt rock or free choice unrefined loose salt – I like to use both. But be sure **not** to provide your horse the traditional refined salt blocks that are intended for cattle and, as previously mentioned, do not feed refined, iodized table salt.

Another concern that arises in equine circles is that a horse will not be able to get enough salt in her diet if she is not consuming "just salt," such as refined table salt or refined salt blocks. Some may apply this same rationale to *unrefined* salt because it contains a small percentage of naturally occurring minerals. There is *no* comparison between unrefined salt and those man-made cattle mineral blocks. That is like comparing apples to oranges. This is another misconception that is leftover baggage from decades of people feeding mineral blocks, as I discussed earlier. Consider it from this standpoint - that line of thinking goes completely against *thousands* of years of time proven unrefined salt consumption. Horses have thrived for millions of years prior to the refinement of salt. So what were horses consuming in order to get their salt ration? You can safely conclude that it *wasn't* refined table salt.

There's been speculation that the reddish salt rocks (i.e. Himalayan or Redmond's) are high in iron and are not a good option to feed insulin resistant (IR) or Cushing's horses. Word got out about this, and many natural hoof care professionals have believed it and gone on to tell their clients not to use what they call "red salts." From my research and observations, I've found that this theory started in a borderline natural equine nutritionist community. That same community recommends refined iodized table salt as well as several other nutritional recommendations for compromised horses that I'd never recommend, nor would I make these same recommendations for healthy horses. It goes without saying (but I'll say it) that I would never follow these recommendations for my personal horses.

For the record, while the statement about iron overload is logical, it's more speculation. What I agree with is that *good* and *bad* sources of iron exist. We have a similar problem with calcium – there's too much *bad* calcium in a horse's diet which leads to calcification in the body. This is *way* more of a problem than the *speculation* of iron overload. My current stance (as of the writing of this book) on the subject of iron overload in horses is this: once objective research has been done on the diet of horses living in the wild and on what are appropriate, healthy, and natural iron levels (and we have a baseline to compare to domestic horses) then you'll have my ear. However, to recommend feeding a toxic, refined salt over a natural unrefined salt to a compromised horse, is irrational.

Additionally, the iron from unrefined salt is in its proper bio-available form along with other balancing minerals – just like nature intended. In my personal experience, I've had no problems with feeding Redmond's or Himalayan salt to my two metabolically-challenged horses. If you're concerned about iron overload due to this speculation, I'd recommend feeding Celtic Sea Salt and be sure to stay away from refined table salt. Celtic does have some iron in it as well, but it's not a "red salt." I've been feeding Celtic Sea Salt and other unrefined salts to my horses for more than 6 years (as of the writing of this book) with nothing but great results. I believe feeding unrefined salt to your horse is one more way to promote a naturally healthy horse.

Another important point is that salt will encourage your horse to drink more water and stay hydrated. This is not only beneficial in hot weather but also in the winter. When its cold, horses are less likely to drink enough water. Appropriate salt consumption helps keep your horse hydrated and decreases the likelihood of her having a colic episode. Water assists the digestive track so it can function in an optimal manner. Colic is more likely to occur during the colder months of the year because a horse may not consume enough water and get enough movement. Additionally, as previously mentioned, the anti-caking agents added to *refined table salt* prevent it from mixing with water. This prevents salt from doing one of its most important functions in the body, which is regulating hydration – another valid reason not to feed refined salt to your horse.

With all that being said, people are becoming more aware of the concept of switching over to unrefined salt. Due to that, more companies are starting to market their own "sea salt" products. Technically all salt comes from the sea in one way or another. Many of these companies are using clever marketing to sell refined salt to you by putting the words "sea salt" on their labels. What they're trying to do is trick you into thinking it is unrefined. So be very careful where you get your salt and make sure to validate that it's unrefined. Refined "sea salt" is just as harmful as "table salt" - they're the same thing. It's just misleading marketing.

One last thing to consider – some people will say feeding unrefined salt is more expensive. I'll leave it up to you to make that judgment. This is how I see it. I do not consider the cost of just the salt. Instead, I consider the cost of all the negative results of using a refined table salt, such as cumulative veterinarian expenses over a period of time, not to mention the lost quality of life and longevity for your horse. All that considered, I don't think table salt is less expensive than unrefined salt at all.

SUMMARY – THE MOST IMPORTANT POINTS TO TAKE AWAY

1. **Salt is critical for your horse.** Do not deprive your horse of salt in her diet. I know of some people who choose not to provide unrefined salt for their horse – either free choice or in their ration. This is a very bad practice and can be detrimental to your horse's health.

2. **Use unrefined salt only.** As I've already discussed, unrefined is the best salt you can provide to your horse. Also, be sure to read all supplement labels, including commercial feed bags and avoid any added refined salt.

3. **Avoid toxins and inappropriate and unnatural substances.** When you have control over it, avoid substances that are not in your horse's best interest – minimize exposure. There are many things we don't have control over, such as breathing in polluted air, but there are ways we can minimize the effects of toxins on the body by

controlling the things we can. In other words, do everything you can to stack the odds in your horse's favor!

4. **Feed a maintenance dose of at least one tablespoon of unrefined sea salt twice per day for an average 1000 pound horse.** It's a good idea to provide your horse at least 2 tablespoons of loose unrefined salt per day (preferably in two separate rations). You may need to add a little more depending on the size of your horse and your weather conditions, but 2 tablespoons for an average size horse is a good baseline.

5. **Provide unrefined sea salt free choice.** When your horse needs it, they will use the free choice option you have in your paddock. Be sure to provide it. We don't always know when our horses may need more nutritional support. Free choice salt will help give them the option of getting the extra nutrients during times when they may need it most. Ideally provide a loose salt option and a lick.

6. **Beware of deceptive marketing.** Be sure to purchase unrefined salt only. Some of the best choices are Celtic, Himalayan, and Redmond's. If the label just says "salt" or "iodized salt" avoid it. As mentioned before, deceptive marketing is often used to promote refined salt under the label "sea salt."

SOURCES FOR SALT

Celtic Sea Salt®
www.selinanaturally.com
www.celticseasalt.com

When you go to purchase Celtic salt for your horse, be sure you purchase the Agricultural/Pet Salt - Celtic Sea Salt® Brand. You can get it in bulk for a reasonable price on Selina Naturally's web site.

Original Himalayan Crystal Salt™
www.thehealingbarn.com
www.hiltonherbs.com
www.himalayancrystalsalt.com

I'd recommend that you be careful of where you get your Himalayan salt. There are some imitations on the market that are cheap sources. A trusted source I use is Hilton Herbs. The Healing Barn is a U.S. distributor of Hilton Herb products. If you are outside the USA you may want to go directly to the Hilton Herbs website to place an order.

Redmond™ Salt

www.redmondequine.com

Redmond provides both loose salt and salt rock for licking. Redmond is a unique trace mineral sea salt supplement that provides the macro and trace minerals your horse needs. They're 100% natural giving your horse nature's perfect blend of minerals. It's harvested from an underground source in Utah – a huge deposit of salt left there from the evaporation of an ancient and pristine sea. It's naturally irregular in shape unlike the chemically processed and compressed square salt blocks.

Icelandic Flake Salt

www.saltverk.com

www.atthemeadow.com

As mentioned previously, this one is more for you to try than to feed to your horse because it's a little pricy. However, if you can find it in bulk for your horse, it would be an optimal choice due to it's higher magnesium content as well as the environmental manner in which it's harvested.

* See the resources section for information on obtaining an element analysis of some of the salts listed .

ADDITIONAL NOTES FROM THE AUTHOR

I hope this book has provided you with some valuable information on salt. I would recommend that in order to get a better understanding of the importance and misconceptions about salt, you read *Salt Your Way to Health*, by David Brownstein as well as dig into the additional resources I've provided for you in this book.

Keep it soulful,
Stephanie Krahl
CEO and co-founder of Soulful Equine

P.S. If you liked this book, you may also enjoy my book *Guiding Principles of Natural Horse Care – Powerful Concepts for a Healthy Horse*. It will provide you with concise and solid information on the emerging subject of natural horse care and answers many common questions about maintaining a naturally healthy horse. To purchase a copy, go to either www.soulfulequine.com or the Amazon web site for your country.

ONLINE RESOURCES

There's an abundance of information available today about caring for your horse naturally. This book was intended to give you another tool in your toolbox for choosing wisely so you can promote your horse's health. The information shared with you in this book is a vital component of a solid natural horse care program. To assist you on learning more about what was discussed in this book and about other aspects of natural horse care, I made a resource area on our website, Soulful Equine. It provides a wealth of information, some of which includes:

> ➢ A list of Soulful Equine articles and reports to enhance your understanding of the concepts discussed in this book.

> ➢ Recommended books, magazines, audios and videos to help further your education on natural horse care.

> ➢ Natural hoof care resources around the web.

> ➢ More on equine dentistry and various other holistic modalities you can look into.

> ➢ Information on putting a non-toxic fly control

program in place that works.

The information contained in these online resources is free to those who buy this book. To request access, go to www.soulfulequine.com and send us an email from the Contact Us page letting us know you purchased this book.

NOTES

1. David Brownstein, M.D., Salt Your Way to Health (West Bloomfield, MI: Medical Alternatives Press, 2006), 75.

2. Mark Bitterman. Salted: A Manifesto on the World's Most Essential Mineral, with Recipes (New York: Ten Speed Press, 2010), 33.

3. Brownstein, op. cit., 27-34.

4. Global Healing Center. "Iodine in Salt: Why Is It Added?" Accessed August 12, 2013. http://www.globalhealingcenter.com/natural-health/iodine-in-salt/.

5. Baseline of Health® Foundation. "A Pillar of Salt." Accessed August 31, 2013. http://www.jonbarron.org/article/pillar-salt.

6. Bitterman, op. cit., 45.

7. Ibid

8. Baseline of Health® Foundation. "Unrefined, Minimally Processed, Non-Iodized Sea Salt." Accessed September 1, 2013. http://www.jonbarron.org/article/unrefined-minimally-processed-non-iodized-sea-salt.

9. Wikipedia. "Erin Brockovich (film)." Accessed August 31, 2013. http://en.wikipedia.org/wiki/Erin_Brockovich _(film).

10. WebMD. "Chromium - Topic Overview." Accessed September 1, 2013. http://www.web-md.com/digestive-disorders/tc/chromium-topic-overview.

11. David Wolfe., The Longevity Now Program (David Wolf, 2010), 123, 288.

12. Beyond the Shaker. "The Death (and Rebirth) of Salt." Accessed August 20, 2013. http://www.beyondtheshaker.com/pages/Salt-Guide-Politics.html#230.

13. Better Than Greens. "Why Celtic Sea Salt? Is There Really Any Difference?" Accessed August 25, 2013. http://www.betterthangreens.com/Celtic-Sea-Salt-Dept/191.

14. Mark Force, DC. "Celtic Salt: The Importance of True Sea Salt." Accessed July 8, 2013. http://drlaurarost.com/Celtic_20Salt.pdf.

15. Brownstein, op. Cit., 75.

16. David Wolfe. 2012 Longevity Now Conference. For more information see: http://www.thelongevitynowconference.com/.

17. Brownstein, op. Cit., 81.

18. Jaime Jackson. Founder – Prevention & Cure the Natural Way. (Harrison, AR: Star Ridge Publishing, 2001), 120.

RESOURCES

Books

- ➤ *Guiding Principles of Natural Horse Care* by Stephanie Krahl, http://www.soulfulequine.com.
- ➤ *Iodine: Why You Need It, Why You Can't Live Without It* by David Brownstein, M.D.
- ➤ *Salt Your Way to Health* by David Brownstein, M.D.
- ➤ *Dr. Jensen's Guide to Body Chemistry & Nutrition* by Bernard Jensen.
- ➤ *Salted: A Manifesto on the World's Most Essential Mineral, with Recipes* by Mark Bitterman.
- ➤ *Salt: A World History* by Mark Kurlansky.
- ➤ *The Story of Salt* by Mark Kurlansky.
- ➤ *Salt Block Cooking: 70 Recipes for Grilling, Chilling, Searing, and Serving on Himalayan Salt Blocks* by Mark Bitterman. This book is the definitive text on Himalayan salt blocks, written by the man who wrote the definitive text on salt.

Recommended Websites

➢ Online resources for books published by Soulful Equine. To request access, go to www.soulfulequine.com and send us an email from the Contact Us page.

➢ Dr. Brownstein's Holistic Medicine. http://www.drbrownstein.com/

➢ Salt Institute - http://www.saltinstitute.org/

➢ Salt News - http://www.saltnews.com/

➢ Selina Naturally – Celtic Sea Salt Brand - http://www.celticseasalt.com/

➢ Redmond Salt - http://www.redmondequine.com/

➢ Dr. Joseph Mercola - http://articles.mercola.com

➢ Salt factoid regarding "salary" - http://en.wikipedia.org/wiki/Salary#Salarium

➢ Dr. Casey Adams, "The Truth About Whole Salt," Healthiertalk.com.

➢ History Quotes - http://www.goodreads.com/quotes/tag/history

➢ Premium Grade Specialty Salts - http://www.saltworks.us/

Articles

All articles accessed from August - September 2013.

➢ *Are You Feeding Your Horse These 4 'Healthy' – Yet Dangerous –Foods?* http://www.soulfulequine.com/feeding-horses-genetically-modified-food/

➤ *Iodine – Getting It Right* by Dr. Lynne August. http://qfac.com/dr-lynn-august-getting-iodine-correct

➤ *High Fructose Corn Syrup: A Sweet and Dangerous Lie.* http://blog.lef.org/2011/11/high-fructose-corn-syrup-dangers.html

➤ *Add This Seasoning to Your Food Daily - Despite What Your Doctor Says.* http://articles.mercola.com/sites/articles/archive/2011/09/20/salt-myth.aspx

➤ *The 9 Foods You Should Never Eat.* http://articles.mercola.com/sites/articles/archive/2013/06/10/9-unhealthy-foods.aspx

➤ *The Guilty Pleasure that Could Save You From Heart Disease.* http://articles.mercola.com/sites/articles/archive/2012/03/05/end-war-on-salt.aspx

➤ *Scientists Officially Link Processed Foods To Autoimmune Disease.* http://www.trueactivist.com/scientists-officially-link-processed-foods-to-autoimmune-disease/comment-page-1/

➤ *Ten reasons why you should use pure unrefined sea salt.* http://www.naturalnews.com/033716_sea_salt_health_benefits.html

➤ *Sea Salt may be Healthier than Table Salt.* http://www.naturalnews.com/025883_salt_sea_body.html

➤ *AMA's campaign against salt fails to recognize health benefits of sea salt and trace minerals.*

http://www.naturalnews.com/019680_excess_s odiu_dietary_salt.html

➤ *Real Salt, Celtic Salt and Himalayan Salt* by Dr. Mark Sircus. http://www.greenmedinfo.com/blog/real-salt-celtic-salt-and-himalayan-salt

➤ *The 13 Amazing Health Benefits of Himalayan Crystal Salt, the Purest Salt on Earth (and Why You Want to Avoid Conventional Salt)* by Dr. Joseph Mercola, http://products.mercola.com/himalayan-salt/

➤ Global Healing Center. *The Harmful Effects of Table Salt.* http://www.globalhealingcenter.com/nutrition/table-salt

➤ Analysis of Natural Himalayan Pink Rock Salt. http://www.saltnews.com/chemical-analys-is-natural-himalayan-pink-salt/

INDEX

ABOUT THE AUTHOR

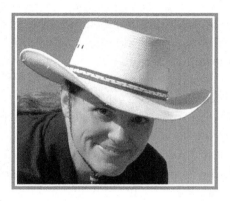

STEPHANIE KRAHL developed a passion for horses at a very young age, and they've played a key role in her life ever since. It started at the age of two with a pony named Thunder, and as a kid she read everything she could get her hands on about horses, from caring for them to learning more about horsemanship.

At the age of nine, with the guidance of her father, she started her first horse under saddle and learned the importance of building a strong relationship with an equine partner.

Her ability to understand and connect with horses

has always been an innate quality. It wasn't until later in life that her education and experience in human health and wellness played a huge role in transitioning her horse care mindset from a traditional to a natural approach. Little did she know that, as a teenager, when a family friend taught her the basics of trimming her own horses, it would come into play later on in Stephanie's life as a natural hoof care provider.

When it comes to horses, Stephanie refuses to settle for mediocre. That passion for learning, and constantly seeking out the best for the horse, has opened up doors far beyond her imagination.

Her degree in Computer Science and Mathematics set up opportunities to become an above average problem solver. Since everything pertaining to horses requires great problem solving skills, it has played a significant role in analyzing, observing and seeking out the best in natural horse care.

Stephanie is a natural horse care specialist, a writer, teacher, coach, CEO and co-founder of Soulful Equine, and author of the book *Guiding Principles of Natural Horse Care*. She teaches horse guardians about natural horse concepts that help their horse *thrive* and regularly provides coaching services as a natural horse care specialist. Stephanie consistently contributes educational articles on natural horse care at www.soulfulequine.com as well as writing for equine publications such as *Natural Horse Magazine* and *Equine Wellness Magazine*.

Other than her passion for horses, Stephanie loves researching and learning about the latest in longevity technologies for both humans and horses, watching movies, staying physically fit, going to the gun range, spending time with loved ones and keeping it soulful.

CONNECT WITH STEPHANIE

www.stephaniekrahl.com
www.soulfulequine.com
twitter.com/soulfulequine
facebook.com/soulfulequine
pinterest.com/soulfulequine

If you want a thriving equine, sign up for Stephanie's email list at:
www.soulfulequine.com.

GET GREAT STUFF FROM SOULFUL EQUINE

DO YOU WANT TO BE NOTIFIED when we release a new book, product, or when we have special discounts?

If so, and if you want a thriving equine partner, then go to the link below to join Soulful Equine's email list.

http://www.soulfulequine.com/email-newsletter/

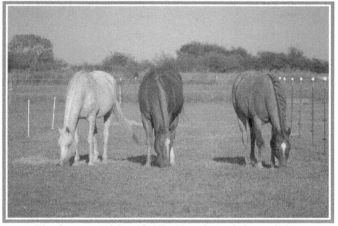

The horses of Soulful Equine from left to right:
Faith, Dillon and Ransom

SOULFUL EQUINE®
Helping Your Horse Thrive™
www.soulfulequine.com

Made in the USA
Las Vegas, NV
25 January 2021

16522868R00049